MORNING PREGNANCY WORKOUT

Easy and Safe Prenatal Exercise Guide

Bonus

Prenatal Affirmation

Alan Hady

TABLE OF CONTENT

INTRODUCTION

Welcoming you to the transformative journey of "Pregnancy workout," this book is a comprehensive guide crafted to illuminate the path of physical well-being during the incredible phase of pregnancy. It is a testament to the harmonious dance between movement and maternity, designed to empower and embrace the holistic benefits that a well-structured exercise routine can offer expectant mothers.

Immerse yourself in a refreshing regimen catered to your shining soul. This book is more than just a handbook; it's a new day for both you and your child.

Consider the gentle stretches, powerful exercises, and contemplative pauses meant to welcome each new day. Say goodbye to exhaustion and hello to the vitality that grows with each carefully managed movement.

This book becomes your valued ally, bringing consolation, strength, and a sense of tranquility. It is written with the expertise of both fitness and maternity professionals.

Join the community of radiant mothers who have turned every dawn into a celebration of life. "Morning Pregnancy Workout" will elevate your pregnancy experience since every morning deserves a tale of energy, and yours begins HERE.

UNDERSTANDING THE MEANING OF PREGNANCY WORKOUT

Pregnancy workout, in the context of this guide, is a deliberate and mindful approach to physical activity tailored to the unique needs of expectant mothers. It goes beyond the conventional notion of exercise, evolving into a celebration of movement that nurtures both the body and the spirit throughout the entire pregnancy journey.

WHY EXERCISE IS IMPORTANT FOR PREGNANT WOMEN

Exercise during pregnancy is not just a recommendation; it is a cornerstone of well-being for expectant mothers. The carefully curated routines in this guide aim to enhance strength, flexibility, and cardiovascular health. Beyond the physical benefits, pregnancy exercise contributes to improved mood, reduced discomfort, better sleep, decreased pain and increased energy levels, fostering a positive pregnancy experience and safe child birth.

WHEN AND WHEN NOT TO EXCERCISE

As much as exercise is important for expectant mothers, it is crucial to understand when not to exercise during pregnancy. If you have any health challenge such as high blood pressure, bleeding, or placenta issue, it is best to see a healthcare practitioner before beginning any exercise plan.

Furthermore, if you feel dizzy, short of breath, bleed, or have stomach discomfort when exercising, you should stop and seek medical attention. To promote a healthy and pleasurable pregnant fitness experience, safety and communication with healthcare specialists is essential.

Try to engage in activities that cause you to feel warm and to breathe more quickly. You should be able to hold a conversation without becoming dizzy or hot, and you should not feel faint or overheated.

GUIDELINES FOR SAFE AND EFFECTIVE EXERCISE

Consult your health care provider before starting any exercise, Listen to your body, stay hydrated, modify as needed, avoid overexertion, monitor your heart rate and wear comfortable clothing.

WORKOUT WITH EMILY

In the chapters that follow, we embark on a journey with Emily, who explores the realms of prenatal fitness, navigates the challenges of each trimester, and embraces the empowering transition to motherhood. Each chapter unfolds a new dimension of the pregnancy exercise experience, offering insights, exercises, and reflections tailored to empower every expectant mother on her unique path.

It is expected that you will have a healthy pregnancy experience and safe delivery, if you adopt the routine carried out by the character in this book at each stage of the pregnancy.

May this book inspire and support you as you embark on the remarkable adventure of nurturing both yourself and the life blossoming within.

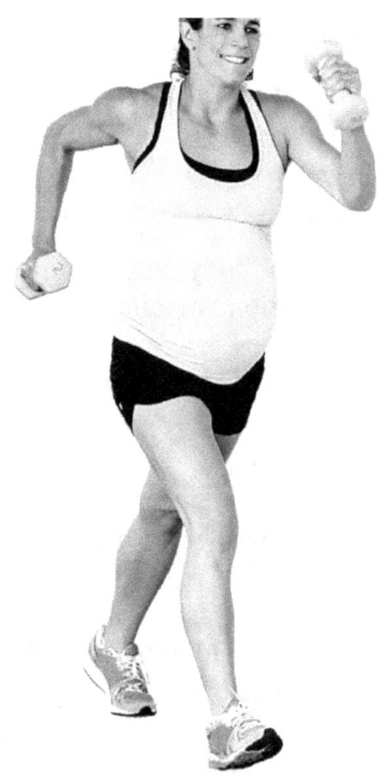

Chapter 1

"DISCOVERING THE MIRACLE WITHIN"

Emily stood in front of the bathroom mirror, her hands trembling as she clutched the plastic stick that held life-altering information. Two pink lines stared back at her, and her heart raced with a mix of excitement and disbelief. Pregnant! The word echoed in her mind, filling the room with an energy that was both thrilling and overwhelming.

As the news settled, Emily found herself on the cusp of a remarkable journey, one that would shape her body and spirit in ways she had never imagined. With the anticipation of motherhood hanging in the air, she made a silent promise to herself and the tiny life growing inside her—a promise to embrace the changes, nurture her well-being, and embark on a path of holistic health.

The decision to prioritize prenatal fitness became the cornerstone of Emily's journey. Amid doctor's appointments and nursery preparations, she recognized the significance of caring for her body to ensure a healthy pregnancy. With a deep breath, she opened the door to a world of exercises tailored for expectant mothers.

The chapter unfolds with Emily diving into the pages of pregnancy exercise guides, absorbing the wisdom of experienced fitness experts and healthcare professionals She discovered the delicate balance between maintaining an active lifestyle and safeguarding the precious life within. From gentle stretches to low-impact cardio, each exercise was a step towards creating a resilient foundation for her pregnancy.

As Emily learned about the benefits of prenatal fitness, the narrative weaves in the voices of other mothers who had embraced similar journeys. Their stories resonated with her, providing a sense of camaraderie and empowerment. The chapter unfolds like a tapestry of shared experiences, illustrating that the path to a healthy pregnancy is both personal and collective.

"Discovering the Miracle Within" becomes more than a chapter title; it becomes a mantra for Emily. The realization that her body is nurturing a new life fills her with awe and gratitude. The chapter concludes with Emily, notebook in hand, jotting down personal fitness goals and affirmations. She closes her eyes, feeling the flutter of life within her, and takes the first steps into a beautiful journey of motherhood, guided by the principles of prenatal fitness.

Chapter 2

"EASING INTO MOTHERHOOD"

Emily's journey into motherhood during the first trimester was akin to a delicate waltz, with each step forward met by the challenges of morning sickness and pervasive fatigue. As the initial excitement settled into the reality of early pregnancy symptoms, Emily embraced the mantra of "Easing into Motherhood," recognizing the need for tailored exercises that would alleviate the discomfort while nurturing her evolving body.

She acknowledged the subtleties of the first trimester—days marked by the unpredictable ebb and flow of nausea and the unexpected bouts of exhaustion. Undeterred, she set out to explore exercises that would become her allies in these moments, aiming to turn the challenges of the first trimester into opportunities for gentle self-care.

Exercise: Mindful Breathing And Seated Stretches

1. ***Mindful Breathing*** (5 minutes): Emily starts her routine by finding a comfortable, quiet space. Sitting cross-legged, she closes her eyes and focuses on her breath. Inhaling deeply through her nose, she allows her belly to expand, embracing the rejuvenating air. Exhaling slowly through her mouth, she releases tension, creating a rhythm that connects her with the present moment.

2. ***Seated Stretches*** (10 minutes): Transitioning into gentle stretches, Emily moves through seated poses designed to alleviate tension in the neck, shoulders, and lower back. With each stretch, she maintains a steady breath, fostering a sense of calm and tranquility. The movements are slow, deliberate, and mindful, promoting flexibility without overexertion.

3. ***Prenatal Yoga Flow*** (15 minutes): Emily engages in a curated sequence of prenatal yoga poses, emphasizing gentle movements that respect the limitations of the first trimester. Supported by modified Downward-Facing Dog, Cat-Cow stretches, and a restorative Child's Pose, the yoga flow encourages a connection between mind, body, and the new life growing within.

4. ***Relaxation and Hydration*** (5 minutes): The session concludes with Emily lying down in a comfortable position, focusing on deep relaxation. She sips on water infused with slices of fresh ginger, a natural remedy for nausea. As she rests, she embraces a moment of serenity, allowing her body to absorb the benefits of the gentle exercises.

With these simple routines, Emily started feeling a renewed sense of energy and connection. Through "Easing into Motherhood," she discovers that adapting exercises to the unique demands of the first trimester not only addresses physical discomfort but also nurtures a positive mindset, setting the stage for a well-supported pregnancy journey

Chapter 3

"STRENGTHENING THE CORE"

With the gentle rhythm of the first-trimester settling, Emily found herself standing at the threshold of a transformative journey. As her body adapted to the intricacies of pregnancy, she recognized the need to build a foundation that would support her throughout the upcoming months. "Strengthening the Core" became a guiding principle, a chapter that unfolded like a roadmap for nurturing the center of her physical strength.

The sensation of growing life within urged her to delve into exercises that would fortify her core—a region undergoing its own set of transformations. As the baby blossomed, so did Emily's determination to cultivate strength and stability in her abdominal muscles.

Exercise: Core-Strengthening Routine

1. ***Pelvic Tilts*** (10 minutes): Emily starts with pelvic tilts, a gentle exercise performed while lying on her back. With her knees bent and feet flat on the floor, she engages her abdominal muscles to tilt her pelvis upward, then relaxes back down. This controlled movement targets the lower abdomen and helps maintain flexibility.
2. ***Seated Belly Breaths*** (5 minutes): Transitioning to a seated position, Emily practices belly breaths. Placing her hands on her growing belly, she inhales deeply, allowing her abdomen to expand. Exhaling slowly, she contracts her

abdominal muscles, fostering a connection with her changing core.

3. *Modified Planks* (15 minutes): Emily moves into a modified plank position, supporting her upper body on her forearms and knees. This exercise engages her core without putting excess strain on her back. Holding the position, she feels a gentle burn, signifying the strengthening of her abdominal muscles.

4. *Side-Lying Leg Lifts* (10 minutes): Lying on her side, Emily performs leg lifts, targeting the oblique. This exercise helps build strength in the lateral muscles while accommodating the changes in her body. The controlled movements contribute to overall core stability.

5. *Gentle Twists* (5 minutes): Incorporating seated or standing gentle twists, Emily promotes flexibility and strength in her core muscles. The twisting motion is performed with mindful breathing, encouraging a sense of balance and tranquility.

6. *Cool Down and Hydration* (5 minutes): The session concludes with a series of gentle

stretches and a focus on hydration. Emily acknowledges the importance of cooling down to prevent muscle tension. She takes a moment to relax, ensuring her body reaps the full benefits of the core-strengthening routine.

With this, Emily felt a newfound sense of empowerment. "Strengthening the Core" becomes a pivotal routine in her pregnancy journey, at this stage, laying the groundwork for physical resilience and a deeper connection with her changing body. As Emily embraces the core-strengthening exercises, she realizes that this chapter is not just about building physical strength but also about cultivating the inner fortitude required for the beautiful journey that lies ahead.

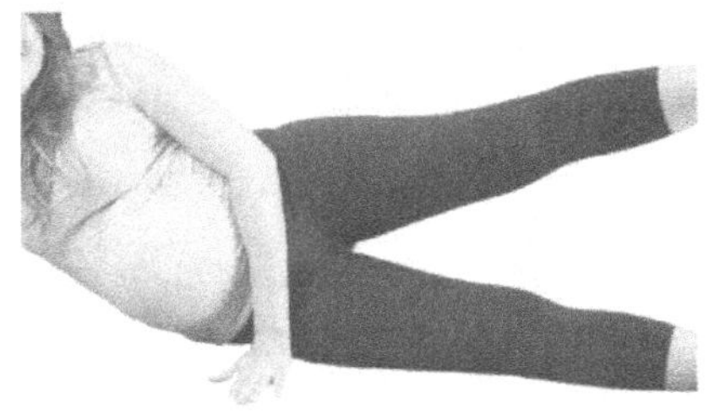

Chapter 4:

"RADIANCE AND MOVEMENT"

As Emily stepped into the second trimester of her pregnancy, a newfound energy radiated within her. The initial challenges of the first trimester began to wane, making way for a sense of vitality and well-being. "Radiance and Movement" became the anthem for this chapter, a celebration of the pregnancy glow and exploration of diverse workouts tailored to enhance flexibility and cardiovascular health.

The chapter unfolds with Emily embracing the changes in her body. The morning sickness and fatigue that characterized the early weeks were replaced by a surge of energy, prompting her to seek exercises that would align with this rejuvenated spirit. As the second trimester unfolded, Emily recognized the importance of movement not just for physical well-being but also for the vibrant glow that seemed to emanate from within.

Exercise: Energizing Second Trimester Routine

1. ***Brisk Walking*** (20 minutes): Emily kicks off her routine with a brisk walk, relishing in the fresh air and the rhythmic cadence of her footsteps. This low-impact cardiovascular exercise not only invigorates her but also sets the tone for emphasizing the benefits of movement during the second trimester.

2. *Prenatal Dance* (15 minutes): Transitioning into a lively prenatal dance session, Emily engages in movements that promote flexibility and elevate her heart rate. The dance routine is designed to be gentle yet dynamic, allowing her to express herself through movement while celebrating the joy of pregnancy.

3. *Swimming* (20 minutes): Emily takes to the water for a refreshing swim. The buoyancy of the water provides gentle resistance, promoting cardiovascular health without putting stress on her joints. As she glides through the pool, Emily revels in the freedom of movement and the soothing sensation of weightlessness.

4. *Prenatal Pilates for Flexibility* (15 minutes): Incorporating a series of prenatal Pilates exercises, Emily focuses on enhancing flexibility while strengthening her core. The controlled movements, combined with intentional breathing, contribute to a sense of balance and suppleness.

5. *Relaxing Cool Down* (10 minutes): Emily takes a moment to connect with her body, acknowledging the symbiotic relationship between movement and the radiant energy she now embodies by concluding the session with a cool-down style, emphasizing stretches that promote flexibility and relaxation

As Emily immerses herself in the diverse workouts of the second trimester, "Radiance and Movement" becomes a testament to the transformative power of exercise during pregnancy.

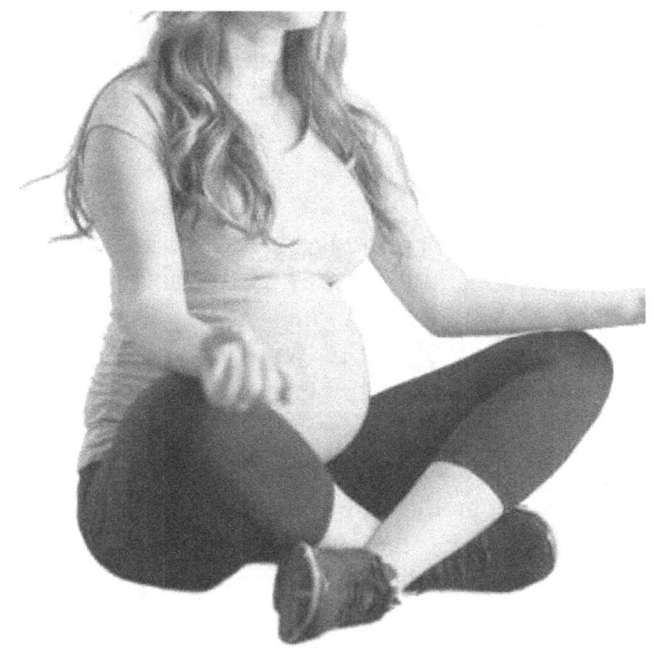

Chapter 5

"CONNECTING WITH YOUR BABY"

In the gentle embrace of the second trimester, Emily felt a profound connection with the life blossoming within her. "Connecting with Your Baby" emerged as a poignant chapter in her pregnancy journey—an exploration of exercises that not only nurtured her physical well-being but also deepened the emotional bond with the tiny soul growing beneath her heart.

The chapter opens with Emily acknowledging the unique bond she shares with her unborn baby. As she contemplates the miracle of life, she embarks on a journey of movement that transcends the physical. It becomes a dance of connection, a rhythmic conversation between mother and child, where every stretch, sway, and breath is a gesture of love.

Exercise: Gentle Bonding Routine

1. ***Mindful Belly Touch*** (5 minutes): Emily begins by finding a quiet space to sit or lie down. Placing her hands on her belly, she takes a few moments for a mindful belly touch. Through gentle strokes and intentional touch, she creates a serene atmosphere for both herself and her baby, fostering a sense of closeness.

2. ***Breathing Yoga*** (10 minutes): Transitioning into a seated position, Emily engages in a breathing meditation. With each inhale, she envisions a flow

of positive energy reaching her baby. As she exhales, she releases any tension or stress, creating a harmonious exchange that transcends the physical realm.

3. ***Partnered Movements*** (15minutes): Enlisting the support of her partner or a friend, Emily explores partnered movements that encourage shared experiences. This may include gentle stretches, synchronized breathing exercises, or even a slow dance—each movement fostering a sense of unity and shared anticipation.

4. ***Water Immersion*** (20minutes): Emily immerses herself in a pool for a water workout designed to enhance both physical and emotional well-being. The buoyancy of the water adds a dimension of weightlessness, creating an environment where she can move freely and feel the subtle response of her baby to the rhythmic motions.

5. ***Guided Visualization*** (10minutes): Emily envisions a serene scene, mentally connecting with her baby in a peaceful environment. This visualization not only offers relaxation but also strengthens the emotional bond, creating a reservoir of positive emotions for both mother and child.

As Emily navigates the exercises in "Connecting with Your Baby," she discovers that this chapter is not just about physical movement—it's a celebration of the profound connection that transcends the boundaries of the womb. The movements become a language, a silent conversation that reaffirms the bond between Emily and her baby, creating a foundation of love and unity that will endure beyond the months of pregnancy.

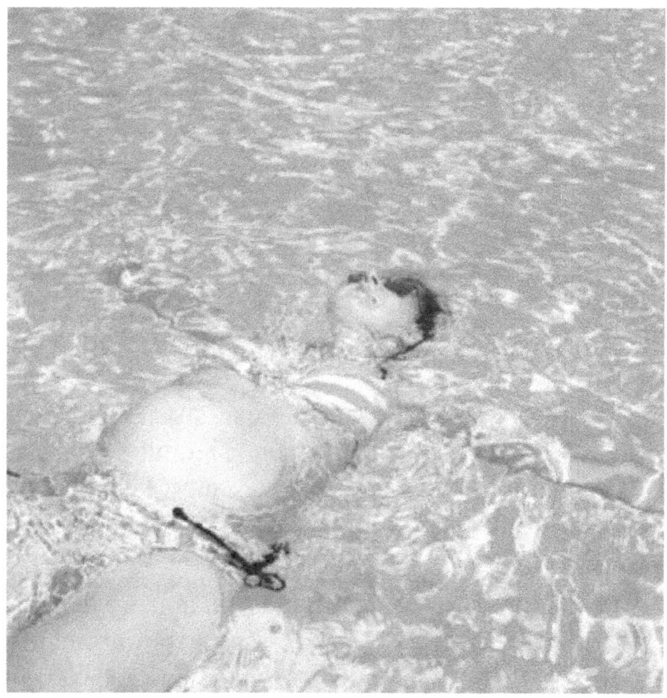

Chapter 6:

"Modifying Workouts for Comfort

With each passing week, Emily found herself on an ever-evolving journey through the tapestry of pregnancy. "Modifying Workouts for Comfort" emerged as a crucial chapter, a guide through the labyrinth of changing needs, and a testament to the art of adapting exercises to ensure both physical well-being and comfort.

Acknowledging the shift in her body, the gentle flutter of life within brought with it a spectrum of changes—some subtle, others more pronounced. As the pregnancy advanced, Emily sought exercises that would embrace the evolving needs of her body, providing both the physical benefits of movement and the comfort essential for a joyful and healthy pregnancy.

Exercise: Tailored Modifications Routine

1. ***Seated Cardio*** (15 minutes): Recognizing the need for low-impact cardio, Emily modifies her routine to include seated exercises. Whether it's seated marches or modified jumping jacks, this adaptation ensures cardiovascular health without compromising comfort.

2. ***Chair Yoga*** (20 minutes): Transitioning into a chair yoga session, Emily discovers the modifying traditional yoga poses. Seated stretches, gentle twists, and modified inversions become a soothing practice, allowing her to embrace the benefits of

yoga while adapting to the changing needs of her body.

3. *Resistance Band Variations* (15 minutes): Emily incorporates resistance bands into her workout, using them for modified strength training. From seated rows to bicep curls, these adaptable bands provide resistance in a way that is both effective and accommodating to her evolving physique.

4. *Prenatal Aquatics* (20 minutes): Embracing the buoyancy of water, Emily explores prenatal aquatics. This water-based workout allows for fluid movements, alleviating any strain on joints and muscles. The adaptability of aquatics proves to be a refreshing and comforting addition to her exercise routine.

5. *Pilates Ball Support* (10 minutes): Utilizing a Pilates ball for support, Emily engages in exercises that strengthen her core and lower body. The ball provides stability while accommodating the changes in her center of gravity, ensuring a workout that is both effective and comfortable.

6. *Mindful Stretching* (10 minutes): The chapter concludes with a session of mindful stretching. Emily focuses on gentle stretches that target key muscle groups, promoting flexibility and relaxation. Each movement is approached with awareness, adapting to the unique needs of her body at this stage of pregnancy.

As Emily navigates the modified workouts, she discovers that the ability to adapt is not a compromise but an empowering choice. "Modifying Workouts for Comfort" becomes a chapter of liberation, allowing her to savor the joy of movement while honoring the changing needs of her body. Through these tailored exercises, Emily realizes that comfort and fitness are not mutually exclusive—they are intertwined elements that harmonize to create a pregnancy journey that is both enriching and uniquely hers.

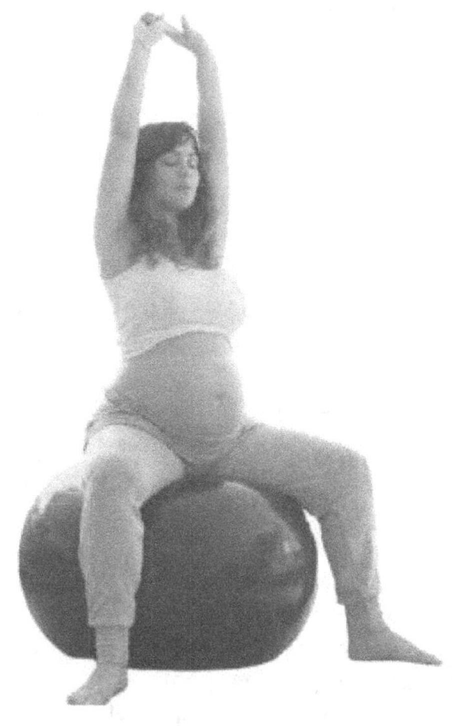

Chapter 7

"Calm amidst the sun"

As the journey through pregnancy continued, Emily found herself seeking a sanctuary within the whirlwind of emotions and physical changes. "Calm Amidst the Storm" unfolded as a chapter devoted to mindful movement—an exploration of techniques that not only nurtured her body but also anchored her mind. In the serenity of this chapter, Emily discovered the profound significance of mental well-being during pregnancy, a journey guided by the soothing embrace of prenatal yoga.

The chapter opens with Emily acknowledging the unique challenges that expecting mothers face—a storm of hormonal fluctuations, emotional shifts, and the physical demands of carrying new life. Recognizing the symbiotic relationship between mental and physical health, Emily set out on a quest for a mindful movement that would provide respite amidst the storm.

Exercise: Prenatal Yoga and Mindfulness Routine

1. ***Breathing Awareness*** (10 minutes): Begin in a comfortable seated position. Close your eyes and bring attention to your breath. Inhale deeply, feeling the rise of your belly, and exhale slowly, allowing tension to melt away. Focus on the natural

rhythm of your breath, fostering a sense of calm and presence.

2. ***Gentle Yoga Poses*** (20 minutes): Transition into a series of gentle prenatal yoga poses. Embrace modified versions of classic poses like. Move with intention, allowing each pose to flow seamlessly into the next. Engage in poses that promote flexibility, strength, and relaxation.

3. ***Mindful Meditation*** (15 minutes): Find a comfortable position for meditation, whether seated or lying down. Guide your attention inward, exploring a mindfulness meditation that encourages a gentle awareness of your body and baby. Allow thoughts to come and go, maintaining a non-judgmental presence.

4. ***Pelvic Floor Exercises*** (10 minutes): Incorporate pelvic floor exercises into your routine. Engage the muscles of the pelvic floor with intention, focusing on both strength and relaxation. These exercises contribute to the well-being of the pelvic region, supporting the physical demands of pregnancy and labor.

5. ***Restorative Yoga*** (15 minutes): Conclude the session with restorative yoga poses. Utilize props such as bolsters and blankets to create a comfortable and supportive environment. Engage in poses like Legs Up the Wall or Supported Child's Pose, promoting relaxation and a sense of surrender.

6. *Affirmations and Reflection* (10 minutes): Take a few moments for affirmations and reflection. Speak words of positivity and love to yourself and your baby. Embrace a sense of gratitude and acknowledge the strength within. Allow the serenity of the practice to resonate within, carrying it into your daily life.

In the tranquil journey of "Calm Amidst the Storm," Emily discovers that mindful movement is not just a physical exercise—it is a sanctuary for the soul. Through the introduction of prenatal yoga and mindfulness techniques, this chapter becomes a beacon of peace, guiding Emily through the intricate dance of pregnancy with a serene heart and a tranquil mind.

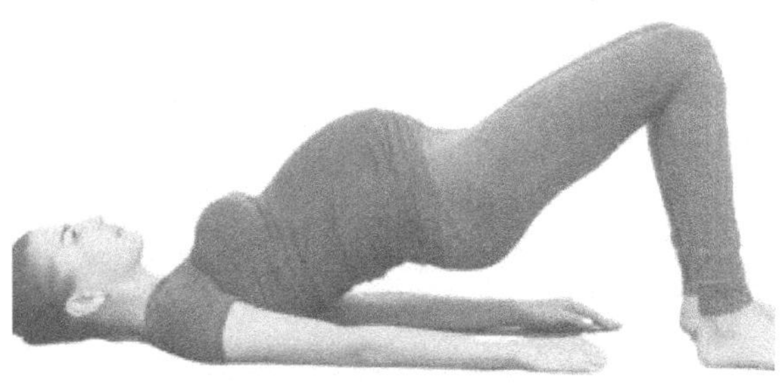

Chapter 8

"Empowering the Body for Birth"

As the countdown to the momentous day of labor and delivery approached, Emily delved into a chapter meticulously crafted for the transformative journey ahead. "Empowering the Body for Birth" unfolded as a guide to fortify the body, mind, and spirit in preparation for the challenges of labor. Through purposeful exercises, Emily embraced the notion that each movement was a step toward empowerment.

The chapter opens with Emily recognizing the impending journey of bringing new life into the world—an endeavor that demands not just courage but also physical resilience. "Empowering the Body for Birth" becomes a mantra, a beacon guiding Emily through a series of workouts designed to enhance endurance, strength, and the vital health of her pelvic floor.

Exercise: Labor-Preparation Workout

Routine

1. ***Prenatal Cardio Conditioning*** (20 minutes): Begin with a session of prenatal cardio designed to elevate your heart rate while being gentle on your joints. Engage in brisk walking, stationary cycling, or modified low-impact aerobics. The goal is to enhance cardiovascular endurance, a crucial component of labor.

2. ***Strength Training for Labor*** (25 minutes):
   Transition into a strength training session tailored to
   the demands of labor. Focus on exercises that target
   major muscle groups, including squats, lunges, and
   modified push-ups. Emphasize controlled
   movements to build strength gradually.

3. ***Pelvic Floor Strengthening*** (15 minutes):
   Dedicate time to specific exercises that enhance
   pelvic floor health. Engage pelvic tilts, and deep
   squats to strengthen the muscles that play a pivotal
   role in labor and delivery. Focus on both strength
   and flexibility for optimal pelvic floor function.

4. ***Yoga for Relaxation and Flexibility*** (20
   minutes): Incorporate a series of prenatal yoga
   poses aimed at promoting relaxation and flexibility.
   Embrace poses such as Child's Pose, Cat-Cow
   stretches, and gentle hip openers. The combination
   of movement and breathwork fosters a sense of
   calm and prepares the body for the challenges
   ahead.

5. ***Endurance-Boosting Exercises*** (20
   minutes): Conclude the routine with endurance-
   boosting exercises. Engage in activities like brisk
   walking, swimming, or stationary cycling to
   simulate the sustained effort required during labor.
   Gradually increase the intensity to challenge your
   endurance levels.

6. _Mindful Cool Down_ (10 minutes): Finish the workout with a mindful cooldown. Incorporate deep stretches and relaxation poses, allowing your body to recover and your mind to find tranquility. Focus on the strength and resilience you've cultivated throughout the session.

In the realm of "Empowering the Body for Birth," Emily discovers that preparation is not just physical—it is a journey of empowerment and self-discovery. Each exercise becomes a testament to the incredible strength within, a resource she will draw upon as she navigates the path of labor and delivery. As the chapter concludes, Emily stands not only physically prepared but also mentally and emotionally fortified, ready to embrace the extraordinary experience that awaits her.

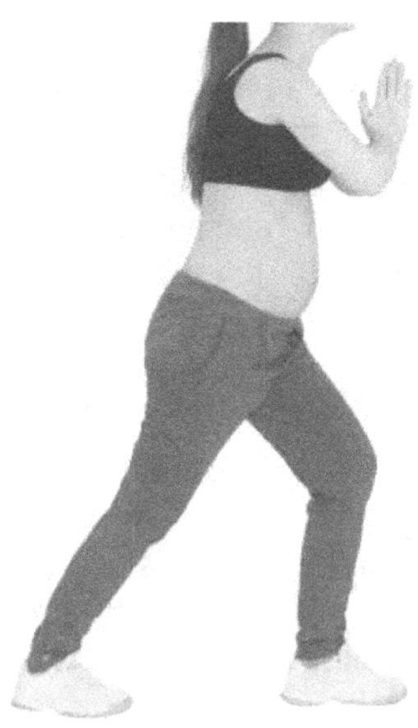

Chapter 9:

"Maintaining Momentum in the Third Trimester

As the final chapters of Emily's pregnancy unfolded, she stood on the threshold of the third trimester—a period of anticipation, growth, and the imminent arrival of new life. "Maintaining Momentum in the Third Trimester" became a pivotal chapter, a roadmap guiding Emily through exercises tailored to ensure a healthy and active conclusion to her remarkable journey.

The chapter opens with Emily acknowledging the unique challenges of the third trimester—a time when the growing belly becomes a testament to the incredible journey within. Yet, in the face of the physical changes and the anticipation of what lies ahead, Emily embraces the concept of maintaining momentum—a commitment to staying active and nurturing her body in preparation for the grand finale.

Exercise: Third Trimester Wellness Routine

1. ***Gentle Cardiovascular Exercise*** (15 minutes): Begin with a session of gentle cardiovascular exercise. Engage in activities like walking, stationary cycling, or swimming to elevate your heart rate while minimizing impact on your joints. The focus is on promoting blood circulation and maintaining cardiovascular health.

2. ***Prenatal Strength Training*** (20 minutes): Transition into a series of strength training exercises modified for the third trimester. Incorporate moves that

target major muscle groups, such as modified squats, bicep curls, and seated leg lifts. Emphasize controlled movements to promote strength and endurance.

3. *Pelvic Floor Exercises* (15 minutes): Dedicate time to specific pelvic floor exercises. Engage in Kegels, pelvic tilts, and gentle stretches to maintain pelvic floor health. These exercises contribute to the overall well-being of the pelvic region, preparing it for the demands of labor.

4. *Prenatal Yoga for Relaxation* (20 minutes): Embrace a session of prenatal yoga focused on relaxation and gentle stretching. Include poses that ease tension in the lower back, hips, and shoulders. Pay attention to your breath, fostering a sense of calm and serenity as you navigate the final weeks of pregnancy.

5. *Low-Impact Endurance* (20 minutes): Conclude the routine with low-impact endurance exercises. Engage in activities like brisk walking or stationary cycling, gradually increasing the duration to challenge your endurance. The goal is to maintain momentum while respecting the limitations of the third trimester.

6. *Mindful Cool Down* (10 minutes): Finish the workout with a mindful cooldown. Incorporate deep stretches and relaxation poses to soothe your muscles and calm your mind. Use this time to connect with your baby and acknowledge the incredible journey you've embarked upon.

As Emily nears the finish line, each movement becomes a celebration, a harmonious dance that brings her closer to the awe-inspiring moment when she will welcome new life into the world.

Chapter 10

"Welcoming Motherhood"

In the grand finale of Emily's extraordinary journey, the final chapter unfurls as a celebration—a tribute to the profound metamorphosis from expecting to embracing motherhood. "Welcoming Motherhood" encapsulates the essence of the entire pregnancy exercise journey, culminating in the holistic benefits of maintaining a fitness routine throughout this transformative period.

Reflecting on the remarkable odyssey Emily has traversed, from the tender discoveries of early pregnancy to the empowering exercises designed for labor preparation, each chapter has woven a tapestry of strength, resilience, and anticipation. As Emily stands on the threshold of motherhood, this concluding chapter becomes a poignant bridge between the chapters of pregnancy and the new beginning awaiting her.

Exercise: Postpartum Wellness Routine

1. *Gentle Postpartum Stretches* (15 minutes): Begin the postpartum wellness routine with gentle stretches. Focus on areas that may have experienced tension during labor, such as the lower back and hips. These soothing stretches aim to restore flexibility and ease any residual discomfort.

2. *Deep Breathing and Relaxation* (20 minutes): Transition into a session of deep breathing and relaxation. Inhale deeply, inviting a

sense of calm and serenity. Exhale slowly, releasing any lingering tension. This practice not only nurtures emotional well-being but also establishes a connection between the new mother and her baby.

3. ***Pelvic Floor Recovery Exercises*** (15 minutes): Dedicate time to pelvic floor recovery exercises. Engage in gentle Kegels and pelvic tilts to gradually restore strength to the pelvic muscles. These exercises contribute to postpartum recovery and promote overall pelvic health.

4. ***Low-Impact Cardio*** (20 minutes): Incorporate low-impact cardio exercises to reawaken the cardiovascular system. Options include brisk walking or stationary cycling, providing a gentle reintroduction to physical activity while respecting the body's postpartum needs.

5. ***Core-Strengthening for Postpartum Wellness*** (20 minutes): Engage in modified core-strengthening exercises suitable for the postpartum period. These exercises focus on rebuilding core strength without putting undue stress on the abdominal muscles. Pay attention to your body's feedback and progress at a comfortable pace.

6. ***Mindful Reflection*** (10 minutes): Conclude the routine with mindful reflection. Take a moment to reflect on the entire pregnancy exercise

journey—from the first steps of discovery to the triumphant culmination of motherhood. Embrace the physical and emotional transformations, recognizing the strength that lies within.

As Emily embraces the transition to motherhood, "Welcoming Motherhood" stands as a testament to the enduring power of maintaining a fitness routine throughout pregnancy. It's not just about physical exercise—it's about cultivating a resilient spirit, fostering a deep connection with one's body, and celebrating the journey that has led to this new beginning. In the tender moments of reflection, Emily finds herself poised at the threshold of a beautiful chapter, ready to embark on the profound adventure of motherhood.

WORKOUT POSE

PELVIS TILTS

Lie on your back with your knees bent. Tilt your pelvis upward, hold for a few seconds, and then return to the beginning position, and repeat the process.

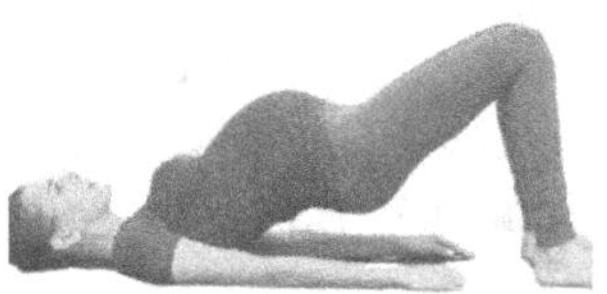

LOW IMPACT CARDIO: WALKING

Take quick walks while maintaining excellent posture.

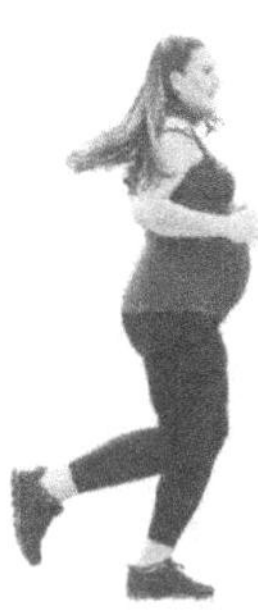

PRENATAL YOGA

Perform mild yoga positions that emphasize deep breathing and flexibility.

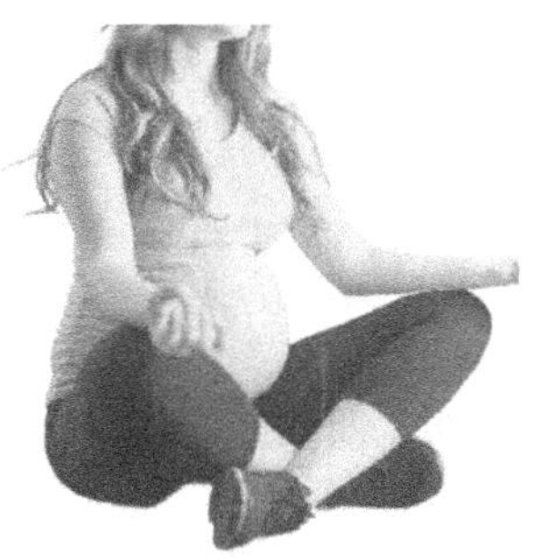

LEG LIFTS WHILE SITTING:

Sit up straight, lift one leg at a time, and hold for a few seconds. Do same to the second leg and repeat.

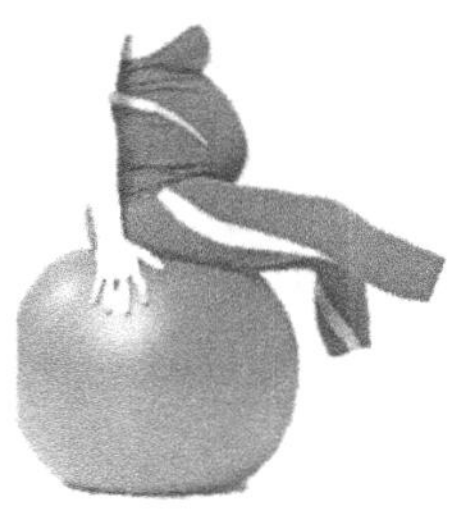

PUSH-UPS AGAINST THE WALL

Place the two palms on the wall, tilt one leg to the back, and do push-ups.

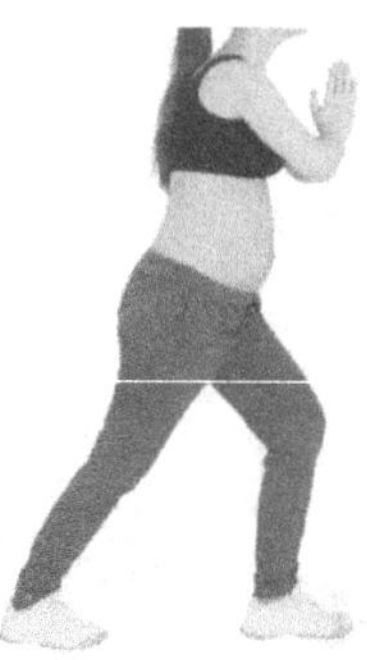

PILATES FOR PREGNANCY

To improve core muscles, focus on controlled movements and repeat the process.

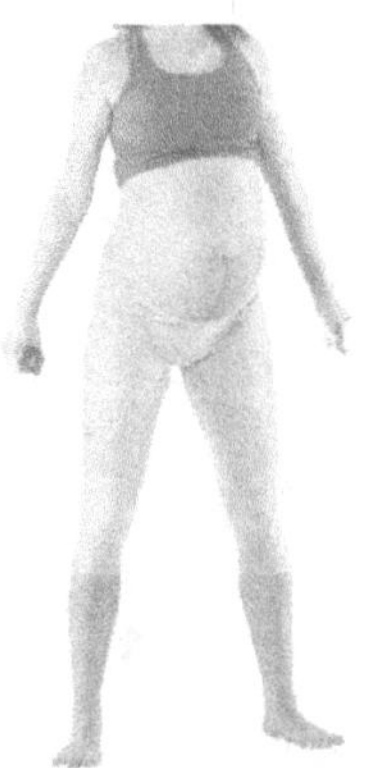

SIDE LYNING LEG LIFT

Lie on your side, lift the upper leg, then slowly lower it, and repeat the process.

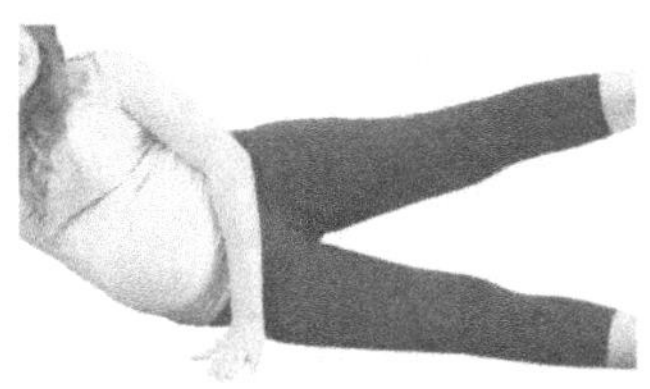

LIGHT WEIGHT BICEP CURLS:

Holding a lightweight in each hand, complete bicep curls with proper posture.

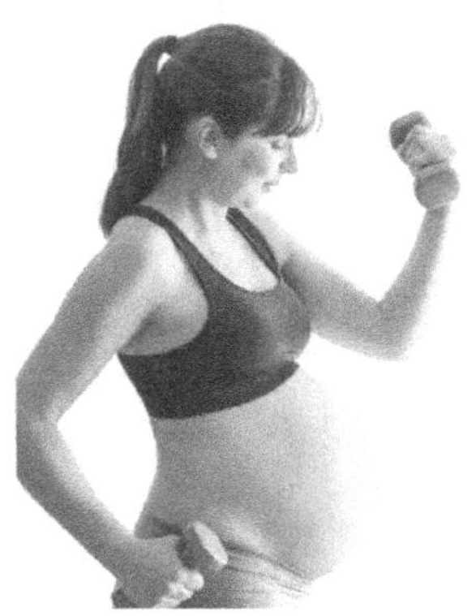

GENTLE SQUAT

Stretch your forearms, set feet hip apart, lower into a gentle squat with or without the help of a ball.

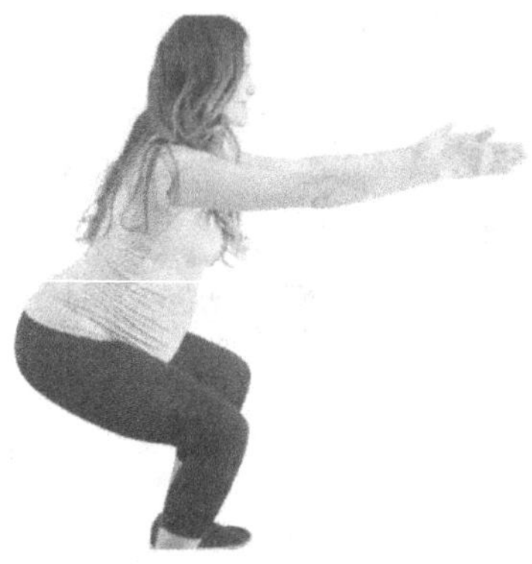

MODIFIED PLANK

Support upper body on forearms and knees

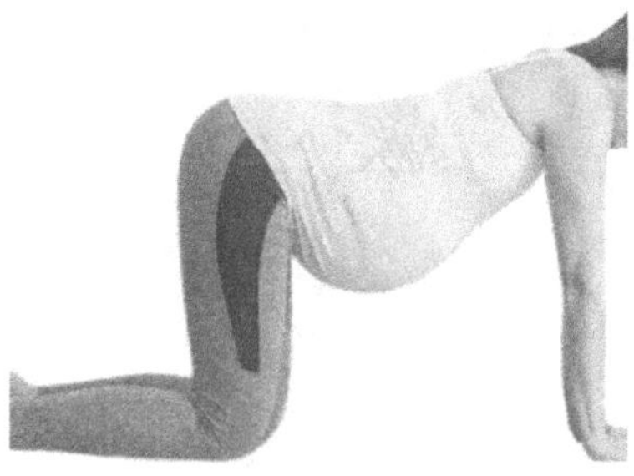

DANCE MOVE

Enjoy pregnancy-specific dancing routines that emphasize soft movements.

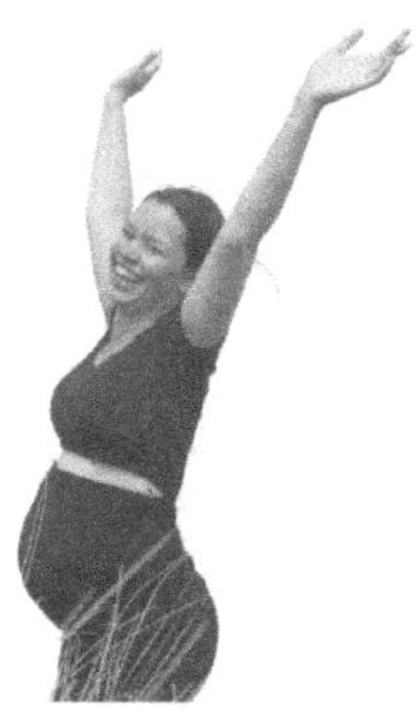

CIRCLES OF THE LEGS:

Lie on your side, raise your upper leg, and make little circles in both directions.

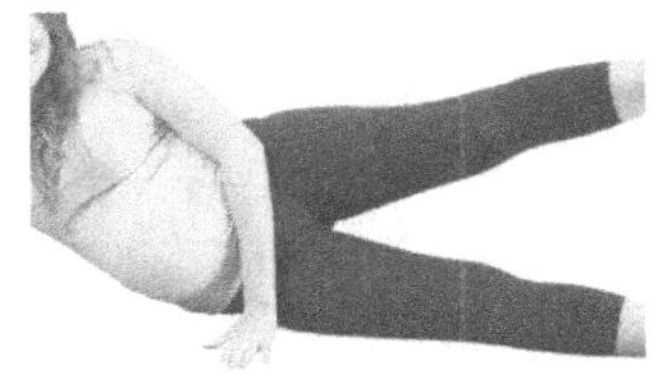

GENTLE STRETCH

 Stretch the main muscle groups while avoiding overexertion.

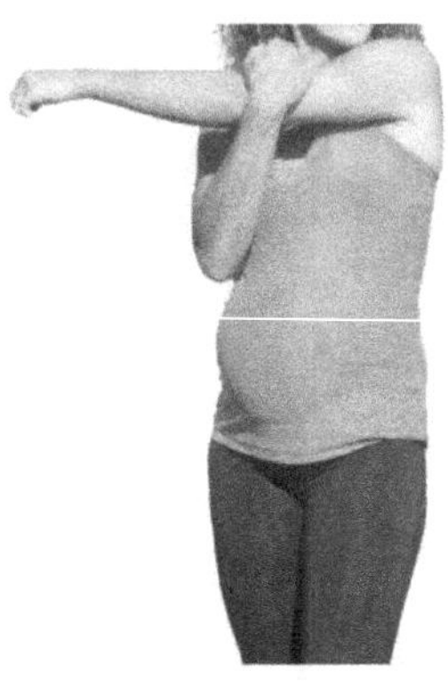

DIPS IN THE TRICEPS:

 Kneel on a flat surface, position your hands on the tummy, and elevate and lower your body.

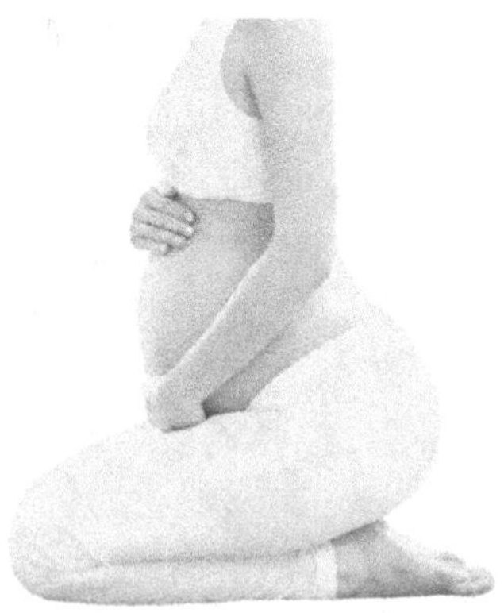

BODY STRETCH USING AN EXERCISE BALL:

 Sit on an exercise ball, raise your hands up, elevate and lower your hands.

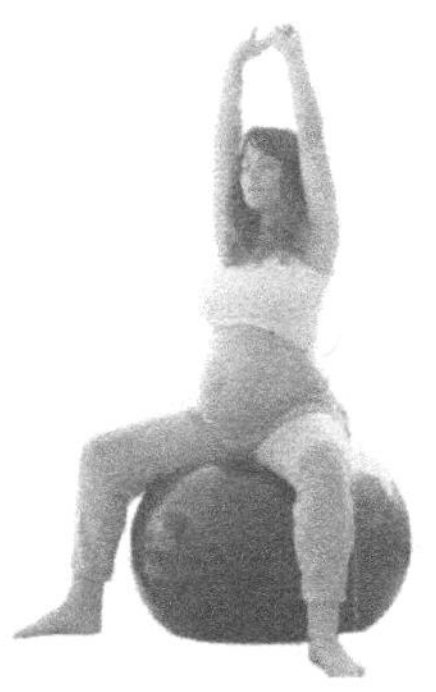

AQUA AEROBICS:

 Swim in a pool and make a gentle turn to promote cardiovascular health.

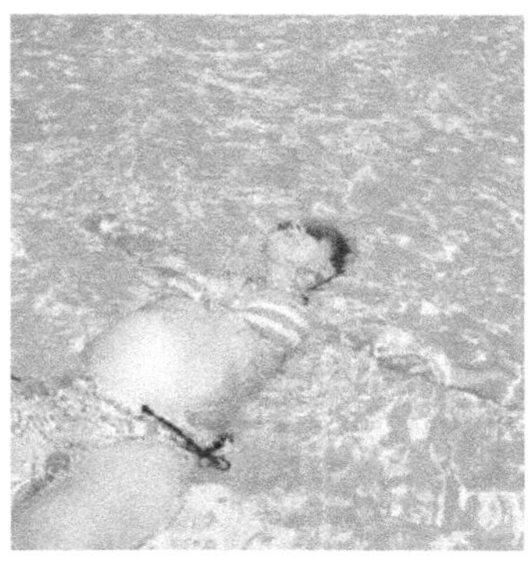

SIDE PLANK MODIFICATION

 Maintain a straight line by supporting your body on one knee, change the knee at intervals, and hold a light weight.

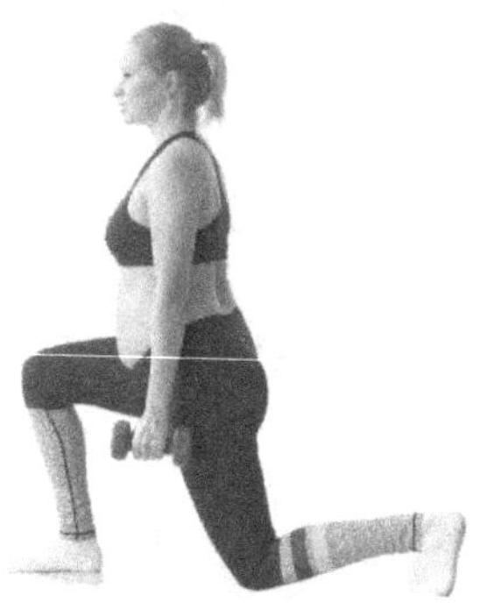

PILATES BALL WORKOUTS

 Sit on a stability ball, make gentle moves, inhale deeply and exhale.

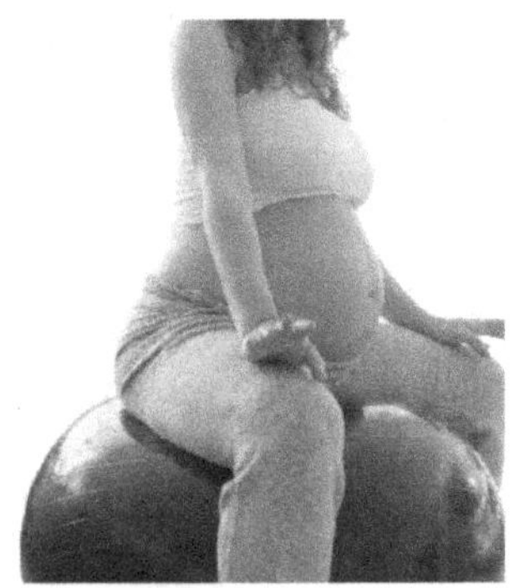

FOREARM PILATE

HOW TO: Kneel down lay the two hands on an exercise ball, and roll it back and forth

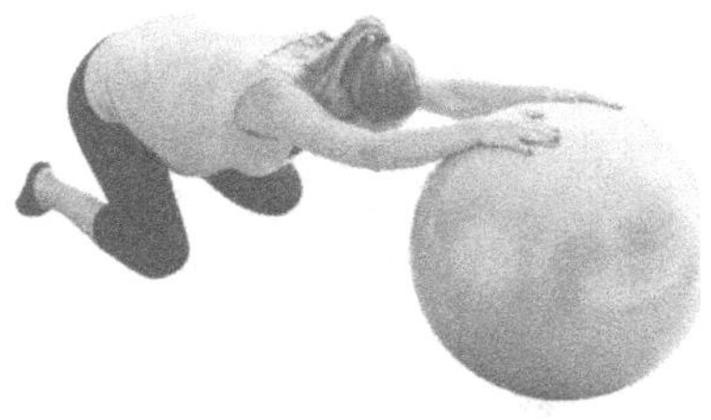

LEG PILATES

HOW TO: Lie on the back, elevate and lay the two legs on an exercise ball, and roll it back and forth.

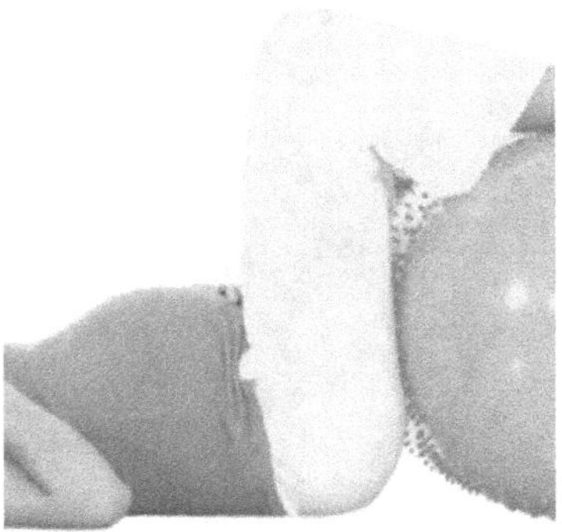

LEG LIFT

Stand upright, palms on the bump, rest the palm of the one foot on the thigh of the second leg, and repeat for the other leg.

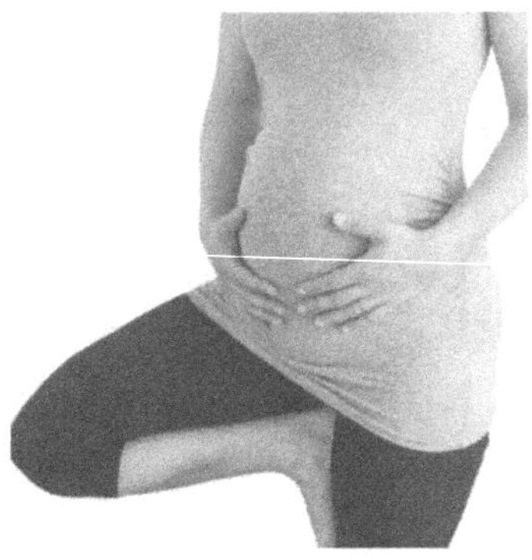

MODIFIED PLANK

Support your body with the elbows and knees, keep back upright and raise one leg at a time

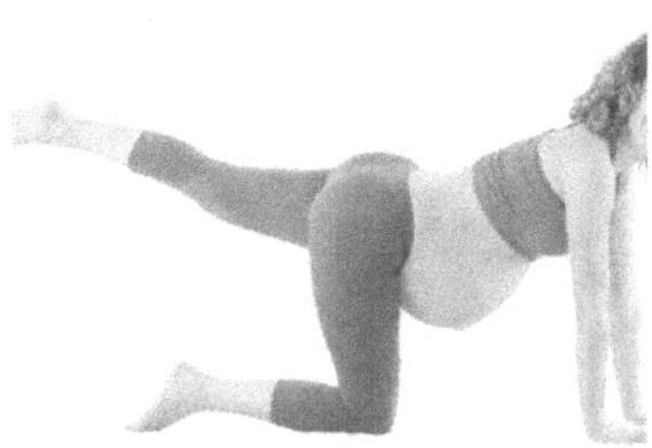

MODIFIED STRETCH

Stretch your two legs apart, straight forward the   two hands to shoulder level and turn the hands sideways.

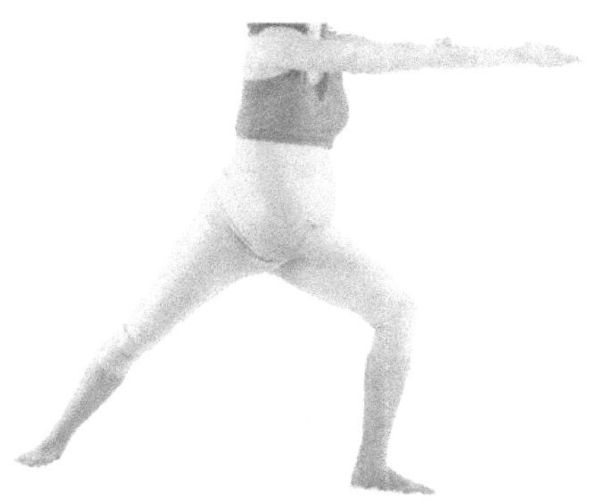

DEEP BREATHING AND RELAXATION

Sit on the two legs, lean backward, gently breathe in and out.

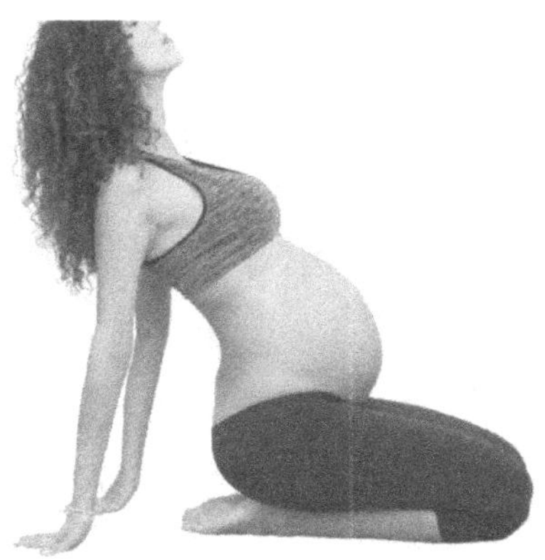

PRENATAL AFFIRMATION

Morning Affirmation:

"With each sunrise, I embrace the gift of a new day. My body is strong, and my spirit is resilient. Today, I choose movement that nourishes both me and my baby."

Midday Empowerment:

"Amid my daily activities, I am mindful of my body. Every step, every stretch, and every breath is a celebration of strength and vitality for myself and my baby."

Afternoon Rejuvenation:

"As the day unfolds, I take moments to pause, breathe, and connect with my baby. My body is a sanctuary, and with each breath, I am filled with tranquility and energy for the exercises ahead."

Pre-Exercise Confidence Boost:

"I approach my pregnancy exercises with confidence and tranquility. Each movement is a dance of empowerment, strengthening both my body and my bond with my growing baby."

During Exercise Positivity:

"In the rhythm of my exercises, I am attuned to the miracle within. With every gentle stretch, I affirm the well-being of my baby.

Post-Exercise Gratitude:

"As I conclude my exercises, I express gratitude to my body for its resilience and to my baby for the shared journey. I am filled with a sense of accomplishment and well-being." Happy new me!

Evening Reflection:

"As the day winds down, I reflect on the beauty of pregnancy. My body is a vessel of life, and I am grateful for the opportunity to nurture and cherish this miraculous journey."

Nighttime relaxation

In the quiet moments before sleep, I affirm relaxation. My body deserves this time to rejuvenate, ensuring a healthy and peaceful night for both of us."

Body Appreciation:

"I appreciate the changes my body is going through. It is a vessel of life, adapting and nurturing, and I honor its strength and beauty."

"Every day, in every way, I am contributing to a healthy pregnancy. My thoughts, actions, and affirmations create an environment of well-being for both me and my baby

End the day with a moment of stillness, acknowledging the power of positive affirmations in fostering a harmonious pregnancy. These affirmations not only shape your mindset but also create an atmosphere of love and positivity for both you and your baby.

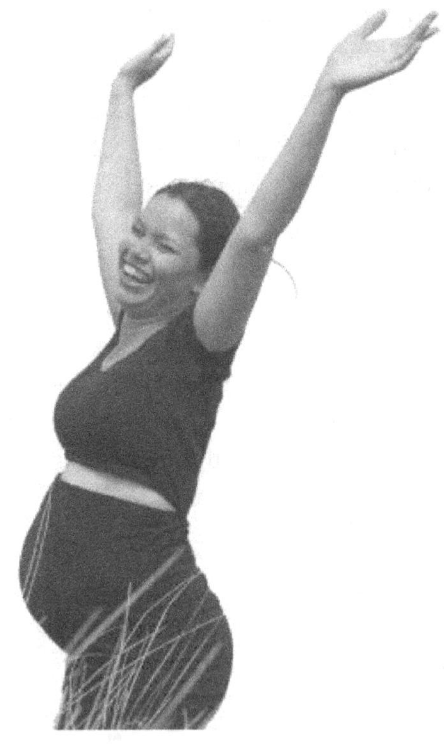

TIPS FOR A HEALTHY PREGNACY AND SAFE DELIVERY

1. Attend prenatal classes regularly to learn about pregnancy, labour and postnatal care monitor both your health and the growth of your baby.

2. Maintain a healthy diet that includes vital nutrients such as folic acid, iron, calcium, and omega-3 fatty acids.

3. Drink lots of water throughout the day to stay hydrated.

4. Engage in safe and moderate exercise regimens appropriate for pregnancy.

5. Prioritize enough sleep to ensure adequate rest throughout pregnancy.

6. To preserve your baby's health, avoid smoking, drinking, and recreational drugs.

7. Maintain frequent checkups to monitor both your health and the growth of your baby.

8. Follow your healthcare provider's recommendations for moderate and healthy weight growth.

9. Pay attention to your posture to avoid back pain and keep your balance.

10. To avoid foodborne infections, avoid raw or undercooked seafood, eggs, and unpasteurized dairy.

11. Educate your birth partner about your plans

12. Make plans for post-partum assistance to smooth the transition and allow for proper healing.

13. Prepare a hospital pack with basics for both you and your infant ahead of time.

14. Wear clothes and shoes that make you comfortable throughout the day.

15. Follow your healthcare provider's advice and instructions

CONCLUSION

As we draw the curtains on the transformative chapters of "Pregnancy Workout," it's not just the end of a book but the beginning of a strong narrative. The journey we've navigated together is not just about physical fitness; it's a celebration of the strength, resilience, and beauty that defines the profound experience of pregnancy.

Consider this conclusion not as an endpoint but as an invitation—a beckoning to continue your journey with the same zeal and commitment. Share this book with fellow mothers, sisters, and friends, for every woman deserves to embark on this transformative pilgrimage. The gift of pregnancy exercise is not just for you—it's for the collective strength of women navigating the beautiful tapestry of motherhood.

In the grand symphony of life, your role is now that of a creator and a nurturer. As you turn the last page, carry with you the wisdom, the strength, and the sheer magnificence of the journey you've embraced. Morning Pregnancy Exercise is more than a book; it's a companion, a guide, and a celebration of the extraordinary journey that is uniquely yours. May your path be filled with vitality, grace, and the unwavering strength that accompanies every woman on her journey to MOTHERHOOD.

Wishing you a safe delivery!

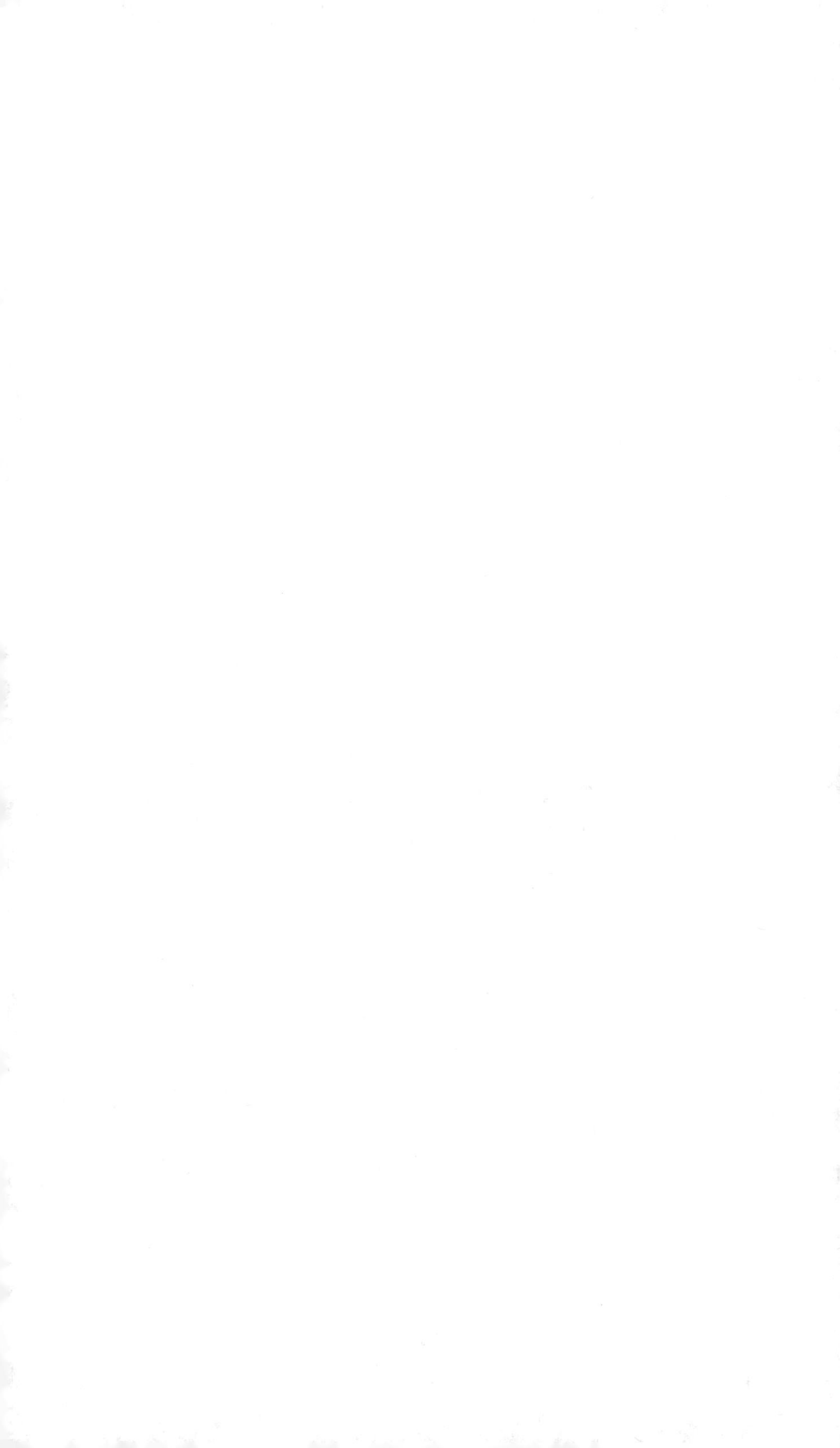

www.ingramcontent.com/pod-product-compliance
Lightning Source LLC
Chambersburg PA
CBHW071117260726

48661CB00006B/2627